FOOD SOLUTION COOKBOOK

A GUIDE TO EATING HEALTHY

DEBRA D. BENSON

DISCLAIMER

TABLE OF CONTENTS

INTRODUCTION

Eating a healthy diet is not about rigid constraints, keeping excessively slim, or depriving yourself of the things you enjoy. Rather, it's about feeling fantastic, having more energy, improving your health, and raising your attitude.

Healthy eating doesn't have to be unnecessarily difficult. If you are overpowered by all the challenging nourishment and meals suggestions out there, you are not the only one. It appears that for every expert who says a specific cuisine is beneficial for you, you'll discover another suggesting precisely the opposite. The fact is that although certain single meals or minerals have been found to have a good influence on mood, it's your overall dietary pattern that is most significant. The cornerstone of a healthy diet should be to replace processed food with genuine food wherever feasible. Eating food that is as near as possible to the way nature created it may make a tremendous impact on the way you think, look, and feel.

Some shopping Recommendations To Get You Started:

* Make a grocery list before you buy and plan what meals you're going to consume.
* Keep the cupboard stocked with items that are fast to prepare and simple to cook.
* Stock up on seasonal veggies, fruit, whole grains, nuts and seeds.
* Choose the reduced fat forms of a product whenever feasible – for example, milk, cheese, yogurt, salad dressings, and gravies.
* Choose lean meat slices and skinless chicken breasts.
* Limit fast meals, chips, crisps, processed meats, pastries, and pies, which all contain substantial levels of fat.
If you have ever wondered about food and how your body utilizes it, then read on.

CHAPTER ONE

WHAT YOU EAT CAN INFLUENCE YOUR HEALTH

Research reveals that food choices increase illness risk. While some foods may promote chronic health issues, others have great therapeutic and preventive benefits.

Thus, many individuals say that food is medicine. Yet, nutrition alone cannot and should not substitute medication in all instances. Although many diseases may be avoided, treated, or even healed by food and lifestyle modifications, many others cannot.

How Food Feeds And Protects Your Body

Many nutrients in food support health and protect your body from sickness.

Consuming adequate, wholesome diets is necessary because their clear ingredients relate reciprocally to create a remark that can not be imitated by taking a tablet.

Vitamins and minerals

Although your body only requires minimal quantities of vitamins and minerals, they're crucial for your health. However, Western diets — high in processed foods and low in natural foods like fresh vegetables — are often weak in vitamins and minerals. Such inadequacies may dramatically raise your risk of illness. For example, low intakes of vitamin C, vitamin D, and folate may hurt your heart, induce immunological dysfunction, and raise your risk of some malignancies, respectively.

Beneficial Plant Compounds

Nutritious foods, including vegetables, fruits, legumes, and grains, feature several beneficial elements, such as antioxidants.

Antioxidants safeguard cells from harm that may cause ailment.

Studies reveal that persons whose diets are high in polyphenol antioxidants have decreased incidences of depression, diabetes, dementia, and heart disease.

Fiber

Fiber is necessary in a wholesome meal . It helps in absorption and evacuation, and also promotes the good bacteria in your abdomen. Thus, high-fiber meals including vegetables, beans, grains, and fruits can guard against illness, lower inflammation, and enhance your immune system.

Protein and Healthful Fats

The protein and fat in full, healthy meals perform different vital functions in your body.

Amino acids – the building blocks of protein — enhance immunological function, muscle synthesis, metabolism, and development, while lipids offer fuel and help absorb nutrients

Omega-3 fatty acids, which are present in foods like fatty fish, help reduce inflammation and are associated with enhanced heart and immune health.

Nutritious Diets Protect Against Disease

Rich diets in plant foods and low in processed items boost your health.

For instance, the Mediterranean diet, which is rich in healthy fats, whole grains, and vegetables, is related to a lower risk of heart disease, neurological diseases, diabetes, some malignancies, and obesity.

Other eating patterns reported to prevent illness include plant-based, whole-food-based, and paleo diet.

Certain diets may reverse some illnesses.

For example, plant-based diets have been reported to reverse coronary artery disease while very-low-carb lifestyles may help remove type 2 diabetes in certain individuals.

What's more, healthier eating patterns like the Mediterranean diet are connected to improved self-reported quality of life and lower rates of depression than standard Western diets – and may even enhance your lifespan.

Can food cure disease?

Some dietary choices may either reduce or raise your illness risk, not all diseases can be avoided or cured via food alone.

Many additional things impact your health and illness risk

Disease risk is highly complicated. Although a bad diet may cause or contribute to diseases, many other variables need to be addressed.

Genetics, stress, pollution, age, illnesses, work dangers, and lifestyle choices — such as lack of exercise, smoking, and alcohol consumption — all have an influence.

Food cannot compensate for bad lifestyle choices, genetic inclination, or other variables connected to illness development.

Though transitioning to a healthy eating pattern might certainly prevent illness, it's vital to remember that food cannot and should not substitute prescription treatments.

Medicine was established to save lives and cure ailments. While it may be overprescribed or exploited as a quick cure for food and lifestyle issues, it's frequently essential.

As recovery does not rest simply on food or lifestyle, opting to skip a potentially life-saving medical therapy to concentrate on nutrition alone may be risky or even deadly.

FOODS WITH HIGH THERAPEUTIC QUALITIES

A good diet may minimize illness risk. Notably, healthy meals may minimize your risk of illness – whereas the converse is true for highly processed diets.

Unhealthy dietary habits may raise illness risk. Unhealthy diets consisting of sugary beverages, fast food, and refined grains are a key contributor to illnesses including heart disease, diabetes, and obesity.

These processed foods destroy your gut flora and cause insulin resistance, chronic inflammation, and overall disease risk.

Transitioning to a diet centered on whole foods may benefit your health in various ways. Foods that have especially significant advantages include:

Berries

Numerous studies have revealed that nutrients and plant components in berries prevent illness. Diets rich in berries may protect against chronic illnesses, including some malignancies.

Cruciferous Veggies

Cruciferous plants like broccoli and kale contain a broad assortment of antioxidants. High consumption of these veggies may minimize your risk of heart disease and enhance your lifespan.

Fatty fish.

Salmon, sardines, and other fatty fish combat inflammation owing to their high quantities of omega-3 fatty acids, which help protect against heart disease.

Mushrooms

Compounds in mushrooms, kinds of which include maitake and reishi, have been proven to enhance your immune system, heart, and brain.

Spices

Turmeric, ginger, cinnamon, and other spices are filled with healthful plant chemicals. For example, studies show that turmeric helps cure arthritis and metabolic syndrome.

Herbs

Herbs like parsley, oregano, rosemary, and sage not only give natural flavor to recipes but also boast several health-promoting elements.

Green Tea

Green tea has been widely explored for its outstanding advantages, which may include decreased inflammation and lower illness risk.

Nuts, seeds, avocados, olive oil, honey, seaweed, and fermented foods are just a few of the many additional foods examined for their therapeutic characteristics.

Simply shifting to a diet rich in natural foods like fruits and vegetables is the easiest approach to receive the medical advantages of food.

A nutrient-dense diet of whole foods has been found to prevent many chronic illnesses and may help treat certain ailments, such as type 2 diabetes.

Although it's apparent that maintaining a nutritious diet is one of the most significant components in living a long, healthy life, bear in mind that you should not depend on food to substitute conventional medicine.

IMPORTANCE OF VARIETY OF FOOD

The value of a variety of food in our diet cannot be emphasized, as it plays a critical part in sustaining general health and well-being. A broad and balanced diet supplies important nutrients, improves digestion, supports immunological function, and adds to the pleasure of meals. Here are some significant reasons showing the relevance of including a diversity of meals in our everyday eating habits:

Nutrient Adequacy

Different diets include varied combinations of vital elements, including vitamins, minerals, proteins, carbs, and fats. Consuming a varied selection of meals helps ensure that our bodies acquire a broad spectrum of nutrients, boosting general health and avoiding nutritional deficiencies.

Disease Prevention

A diversified diet has been connected with a lower risk of chronic illnesses, including heart disease, diabetes, and some malignancies. Different foods include distinct bioactive chemicals and antioxidants that contribute to the body's defense against oxidative stress and inflammation, crucial elements in disease prevention.

Gut Health

A diversified diet is helpful for gut health. The millions of bacteria in the digestive system thrive on a range of fibers and minerals. A varied variety of meals fosters the formation of a healthy microbiome, which is associated with improved digestion, greater nutrient absorption, and a stronger immune system.

Weight Control

Including a variety of foods in your diet will aid with weight control. Different foods have varied degrees of satiety, meaning they may make you feel full and satisfied. A balanced diet with a mix of proteins, fats, and carbs may lead to improved hunger control and weight management.

Culinary Enjoyment

Variety in food increases the sensory experience of eating. It reduces monotony, stimulates the taste, and makes meals more delightful. Trying different tastes, textures, and cuisines adds excitement to the eating experience, developing a good connection with food.

Cultural Appreciation

Embracing a range of meals helps people to understand and appreciate diverse civilizations via their culinary traditions. It encourages diversity and understanding, as well as a feeling of connectedness to the global community via shared eating experiences.

Environmental Sustainability

Diversifying our dietary choices may help with environmental sustainability. By adopting a range of plant-based meals and lowering dependence on a few staple crops or animal products, we may promote more sustainable agriculture methods and help alleviate the environmental effects of food production.

Psychological Well-Being

Food is not only nourishment for the body but also has a major influence on mental and emotional well-being. Enjoying a variety of meals may lead to a healthy connection with food, minimizing the chance of restricted eating habits or disordered eating behaviors.

Adaptability to Lifestyle Changes

Life circumstances, such as age, activity level, and health issues, may demand adaptations to dietary requirements. A diversified diet gives flexibility, making it simpler to adjust to changing nutritional needs during various phases of life.

CHAPTER TWO
HEALTHY EATING HABITS

Eating properly involves adopting a healthy eating pattern that includes a range of nutritional meals and fluids. It also implies receiving the quantity of calories that's ideal for you (not eating too much or too little).

Healthy eating habits are crucial as far as food is concerned. The quality and amount of foodstuff, for the well-being of the consumer and the eaten. Eating the proper quantity and the highest quality of food delivers the ideal healthy state. The correct quality of food comprises various food ingredients.

The amount of food required by a person, however, varies on different circumstances. Consuming too much food is not only bad for human health but also for the ecosystem. The highly exploited plants may potentially experience the danger of extinction.

Below are guidelines you need to implement to have a healthy eating habit

1. Prepare meals from scratch

Preparing your meal with fresh ingredients helps you to look out for sodium, sugar, and fat levels, which is hard to look out for when you buy prepared food. Preparing meals at home is also cheaper than eating out. Besides ensuring that you obtain appropriate nourishment, cooking meals from whole foods may also improve your mood, according to certain research.

2. Eat Smaller Servings

Restaurant servings are sometimes adequate for two or three individuals. Control your portion size by ordering an appetizer or a small plate instead of an entrée, or by sharing an entree with a buddy. At home, serve meals on tiny plates, which might make your quantity seem bigger. Studies have revealed that individuals are more inclined to overeat when they are eating from bigger plates.

3. Avoid Sugary Beverages (especially fruit juice)

Daily intake of sugary beverages such as soda and fruit juice raises the risk of obesity, type 2 diabetes, and heart disease. In addition, the fructose in these beverages does not make the body feel full, thus soda consumers tend to take more total calories than people who do not drink soda.

4. Enjoy Coffee (not much and without sugar)

Coffee intake is connected with a decreased risk of type 2 diabetes, and may be associated with a lower risk of dementia and Alzheimer's, however adding sugar may counteract some of the health advantages. While drinking too much coffee may induce anxiety and sleeplessness in certain individuals - mostly dependent on heredity – a recent ingesting three to four cups of coffee in a day may have health issues and advantages

5. Plan meals and prepare extra for leftovers

Meal planning will help you keep an eye on nutrients and can guarantee you are eating a well-balanced diet. Plan a couple of dinners a week around dishes you and your family enjoy and buy for those items. It seems like a no-brainer, but how many times have you been caught hungry with an empty fridge and ended up ordering delivery or going out to eat? Prepare food that will remain for days, so that you can cook twice a week.

6. Manage your intestines health with grain and bacteria

The bacterial colony in your intestines, termed your gut microbiota, is tied to your mood, immune system, and susceptibility to chronic inflammatory disorders and obesity. Two wonderful strategies to maintain your microbiota health include consuming adequate dietary fiber and eating probiotics, either in the form of dietary supplements containing active cultures or by eating fermented foods such as yogurt and sauerkraut.

7. Don't dread all fats

The assumption that consuming fat makes you fat is antiquated. Your body requires fat to operate and absorb nutrients, and critical fatty acids, notably omega-3s, are necessary for normal brain function. Unsaturated fats, such as those found in olive oil, nuts, seeds, seafood, and avocados are considered beneficial. The idea is to avoid trans fats and minimize saturated fat consumption.

8. Eat more whole fruits and vegetables

A diet heavy in fruits and vegetables is connected with decreased risks of cancer, heart disease, stroke, and diabetes. Recent research also reveals that eating more fruits and vegetables may help psychological health as well.

9. Drink water, particularly before meals

The necessity of drinking water cannot be emphasized. It maintains the kidneys working — and helps avoid kidney stones – while also reducing constipation and dehydration. It is also connected with weight control. Replacing sugary beverages such as soda with water may lead to a lower calorie intake, and some research shows that those who drink water before meals may eat fewer calories and also lose weight more rapidly.

10. Consider nutrition instead of calculating calories

Reducing everyday eating habits to a calorie count misses the reality that many meals offer empty calories with little nutritional benefit. Some meal selections have a large quantity of nutrients per ounce and are more satiating, which may help you eat fewer calories at the end of the day. Take nuts for example: They include fiber, which helps you feel full instantly, and protein, which helps you feel full

for longer. Rather than tracking calories, concentrate on consuming high-quality meals such as whole grains, veggies, and healthy protein sources.

11. Eat a range of proteins

Protein is vital to any diet, and happily, proteins are simple to acquire from animal and plant sources. Proteins are produced from amino acids, and nine of them – termed essential amino acids – are the ones that the human body cannot manufacture and must take from food. Eating a variety of plant protein sources, including legumes, nuts, seeds, and whole grains may deliver the entire spectrum of these important amino acids. Poultry, fish, and eggs are regarded to be better animal sources of protein than red meat and dairy.

12. Eat less salt

High salt consumption may contribute to high blood pressure and heart disease. Because most of the salt we swallow comes from commercially produced foods, as opposed to home-cooked meals, it is crucial to read labels on pre-packaged items and monitor sodium consumption. The major sources of salt in American diets include bread, pizza, savory snacks such as potato chips and crackers, sandwiches, cured meats including lunch meat, soups, tacos and burritos, eggs, poultry, and cheese.

13. Eat Egg but not in excess

Eggs are a nutrient-dense protein source. Many studies have demonstrated that eating up to one egg a day is not connected with an increased risk of heart disease in healthy persons who are not diabetic. A 2019 research, however, demonstrates a connection between increased intake of dietary cholesterol, especially eggs, and a higher incidence of coronary heart disease. This risk was connected to consuming, on top of a typical diet, three to four eggs or 300 mg of dietary cholesterol per week.

14. Instead of processed food, nibble on almonds

Keeping a jar of nuts in your vehicle or pocket may help minimize harmful snack purchases and potentially lessen the chance of weight gain. Recent research reveals that frequently nibbling on small quantities of nuts may prevent excessive weight gain and lessen the risk of obesity. Nuts provide protein, fiber, and healthy fats, all of which help you feel full for longer.

15. Consume fatty fish

It is suggested to take two meals of fish – preferably fatty fish such as sardines, salmon, herring, albacore tuna, and lake trout – every week. These fish are abundant in protein as well as omega-3s, which contribute to heart health.

16. Limit high-glycemic index foods

Although all carbs are turned into glucose in the body, some are processed considerably quicker than others, causing blood sugar levels to surge. The glycemic index grades carbohydrates on how fast and how much they raise blood sugar levels. Eating high-glycemic meals such as white bread and refined sugars may raise your risk of type 2 diabetes and heart disease. Foods that are abundant in fiber, such as whole grains, broccoli, beans, and apples with their peel take longer to digest and consequently, the converted sugar is released slowly into the blood. Foods having their fiber removed, such as white flour, are higher on the glycemic index.

17. Use more fresh herbs

Not only is using fresh herbs a simple and affordable way to make regular cuisine exciting, but it is also a terrific method to enhance your nutritional intake. Leafy herbs such as dill, parsley, and basil are nutritionally comparable to other leafy greens, such as spinach, and may include vitamins A, C, and K. While herbs are commonly used dried in tiny amounts as a spice, they may also be utilized fresh in huge quantities. Try adding chopped chives to an omelet, heaping cilantro on tacos, or tossing a handful of fresh basil into soup before serving.

18. Pay attention to your body

How frequently do you feel fatigued or have an upset stomach after eating? Stress, multitasking while eating, having a food sensitivity, or not digesting food fully may all contribute to indigestion or discomfort. Notice how you feel after you eat. Do some meals always irritate your stomach? If so, you may need to obtain an allergy test. The first step toward healthy digestion is just recognizing what occurs in your body after you eat.

19. Ensure you're receiving enough vitamin D

Vitamin D is vital to bone health, and lack may be related to increased risk of heart disease and cancer. Dietary sources include some fish and fish liver oils, egg yolks, UV-treated mushrooms, and fortified dairy and cereals.

20. Keep nutritious foods at home, so you don't seek bad foods

Consuming unhealthy food alternatives may be more impactful than good ones. It is a good idea to have healthy meals stocked and avoid bringing home bad food. A bowl of fruit, veggies, hummus, or a container of almonds within easy reach may healthily meet snacking desires.

21. Eat whole grains

A diet rich in whole grains may minimize the incidence of heart disease and diabetes. Unlike processed grains whose bran and germ have been removed, whole grains maintain their fiber and minerals. Fiber helps delay the digestion of carbohydrates, which avoids abrupt rises in blood sugar. Cooking using unprocessed whole grains such as amaranth, barley, oats, and wild rice helps guarantee you obtain more of the nutrients that these grains provide.

22. Reduce red meat intake, particularly processed meats

Although rising research shows that we should restrict our diet of red meat – particularly processed red meat – many people still enjoy burgers and sausages. If you're going to consume red meat, avoid processed and cured meats such as ham, lunch meat, and bacon, since they may be related to cancer and heart disease. Instead, consider lean, unprocessed grass-fed beef, which is richer in omega-3 fatty acids. While accessible to relatively few people, wild game such as elk, venison, or bison, which tend to be lower in saturated fats than farm-raised animals, is another better alternative.

23. Don't diet or consider items as "off limits"

Restricted eating (dieting) may actually induce individuals to overeat and concentrate on their hunger. Dieters who heard two-sided messages, however, focused on both the good and bad elements of the meal, were more likely to pick less harmful items.

24. Sub homemade popcorn for potato chips

Chips tend to be higher in fat and calories than popcorn unless the popcorn is the microwaved, butter-flavored sort. Choose air-popped corn for a whole-grain, fiber-packed snack that you can eat by the handful. It takes around six cups of popcorn to get the same amount of calories as one cup of chips.

25. Make little adjustments, one step at a time

Several studies show that adopting incremental modifications in food and lifestyle may be more beneficial and durable than abrupt dramatic alterations. Instead of adopting a severe fad diet, establish tiny, achievable objectives like eating one additional piece of fruit every day.

Benefits of Eating Healthy Food

A well-balanced diet gives you all of the energy you need to be active throughout the day and nutrients you need for development and repair, enabling you to stay strong and healthy and help to avoid diet-related sickness, such as certain cancers.

Keeping active and eating a healthy balanced diet will also assist you in maintaining a healthy weight.

Benefits

- Type 2 Diabetes

Maintaining a healthy weight and eating a balanced diet that's low in saturated fat and rich in fiber found in whole grains will help to minimize your chances of getting type 2 diabetes.

- Heart Health

A balanced diet rich in fruits, vegetables, whole grains, and low-fat dairy may help to minimize your risk of heart disease by managing blood pressure and cholesterol levels.

High blood pressure and cholesterol might be a result of too much salt and saturated fats in your diet.

- Strong bones and teeth

A meal that contains enough calcium helps your teeth and bones to be strong and also helps to reduce bone loss. You can gain enough calcium when you consume:

dark green vegetables – such as kale and broccoli, calcium-braced meals like soya produce, fruit juices and barley.

As vitamin D helps your body absorb calcium, make sure you get outside (your body gets vitamin D from the sun) and have plenty of foods containing vitamin D in your meals like oily fish and braced barley.

RIGHT EATING STARTS IN THE GUT

Digestive system disorders are widespread and produce symptoms such as gas, heartburn, bloating, and constipation. A multitude of variables may affect digestive system health, including aging and other health issues. Eating for your gut is one crucial approach to enhance digestive health and avoid symptoms.

Making healthier food choices requires eating a balanced diet that is rich in fruits and vegetables. These meals supply the fiber required to produce beneficial bacteria and defend intestinal health. In general, preferring natural meals over processed ones will support good digestion. Processed foods frequently have additional sugar, fat, and salt. In addition, processed foods may have lost many of their natural nutrients throughout the food production process.

Here are five meals that promote healthy digestion and help you avoid typical stomach issues:

1. Whole Grains

White or brown rice? Whole-wheat or white bread? Doctors recommend that if you want your gut to operate better, consider whole grains, as healthy colon function needs at least 25 grams of fiber daily. Compared to processed carbs, like white bread and pasta, whole grains give tons of fiber, as well as extra nutrients, such as omega-3 fatty acids. When gut bacteria digest fiber, they generate short-chain fatty acids. These substances stimulate appropriate activity in the cells lining the colon, where 70 percent of our immune cells exist.

Despite the popularity of low-carb diets for weight management, skipping grains completely may not be so helpful for the healthy gut flora that thrives on fiber.

2. Leafy Greens

Leafy greens, such as spinach or kale, are good providers of fiber, as well as minerals including folate, vitamin C, vitamin K, and vitamin A. Research suggests that leafy greens also contain a special sort of sugar that helps stimulate the development of beneficial gut flora.

Eating a lot of fiber and leafy greens assists you in creating a perfect gut microbiota – those billions of organisms that reside in the colon.

3. Lean Protein

People with IBS or gastrointestinal sensitivity should stay with lean proteins and avoid meals that are heavy in fat, particularly fried dishes.

High-fat diets may stimulate contractions of the colon, and the high-fat content of red meat is only one reason to pick healthier choices. Experts suggest that red meat also encourages intestinal bacteria that generate compounds connected with an increased risk of blocked arteries.

4. Low-Fructose Fruits

If you're someone who's prone to gas and bloating, you may want to consider limiting your intake of fructose, or fruit sugar. Some fruits such as apples, pears, and mango are all rich in fructose.

On the other side, berries and citrus fruits, such as oranges and grapefruit, contain less fructose, making them easier to stomach and less prone to create gas.

CHAPTER THREE

ESSENCE AND CONCEPTS OF SEPARATE NUTRITION

Individual nutrition's notion is built on the individual usage of products that were incompatible. The confirmed truth explains this strategy that for digesting distinct forms of food, issues that are diverse, are required. If one form of food enters your body, are you as efficient as you are able to, which substantially promotes digestion and further digestion of materials? The game of nutrients drops slightly, which leads to interruptions within the digesting method whenever a combination meal is associated with it. Consequently, food that is natural begins to ferment and starts to get transferred within the sort of products and fats, intoxicating metabolism, and your body decelerates.

Based on the program of individual food – all food may be split into three basic teams: meals comprising predominantly carbohydrates, protein meals, and natural meals (veggies, blueberries, herbs, fruits, etc.). The very first two teams are absolutely incompatible with one another, food in the team that was next might be matched with others with these.

Concepts of Individual Diet

Additionally, you may still discover certain principles of individual diet, which demand adherence that is necessary. To begin with, you need to keep to the interval between your methods of goods that are incompatible; its duration must absolutely be three hours or at least two. It's essential merely when eating isn't recommended when you have a true sense of starving. The intake of water may begin four hours following the protein items, and a couple of after the intake of meals including carbohydrates. Additionally from drinking it's encouraged to abstain for five before eating for fifteen minutes. The belly shouldn't be packed fully. Consume gently, delicately moistening with eating and spit on food.

Provide options for the simple meals uncommon for your location. It's appealing that the majority of it is not placed through heat treatment to safeguard all useful materials. Raw foods must absolutely constitute at least 2% of the ration. Meals for individual meals must surely be arranged from the approach to cooking or boiling. At the same time, similarly prepared and uncooked food must have a heat that is pleasant.

BUILDING A HEALTHY - GIVING PANTRY

Having a well-stocked pantry is one of the finest ways you can set yourself up for success in the kitchen. Not only does having nutritious foods on hand provide for simple, evening dinners, but it also minimizes stress surrounding "what's for dinner". You'll also save you time and money!

But I understand it! It might be hard to know how to start, what to have on hand, and how to utilize it. I hope this essay helps you feel confident about how to fill your kitchen with pantry necessities. This list will offer you a basis for producing nutritious, balanced meals. From there, you may incorporate fresh fruit and proteins into your weekly cycle.

How to Stock a Healthy Pantry

Pantry staples might imply various things to different individuals. For me, this includes goods you can keep in the pantry, fridge, and freezer that will remain fresh for at least two weeks. Think plant-based proteins like beans and lentils, nuts, seeds, and longer-lasting veggies. This ensures that you have a range of foods and may build a balanced meal that contains protein, healthy fats, fiber-rich carbs, and veggies. Think of the pantry basics as the key components of your meals. From there you may add in fresh veggies or proteins, as required.

- Pantry Purge

Before you start out to replenish your pantry, you need to clear it out. Go through your pantry, fridge, and freezer products and trash anything that's outdated or you simply don't use. Now is the time to tidy up your selections. Toss or donate any highly processed food with large ingredient lists and/or ingredients you don't recognize. Think of your pantry cleanout as a blank slate. Getting rid of these ultra-processed items provides a way for nutritious, genuine food.

- Take Inventory

Now it's time to do an inventory. Once you've cleared away the highly processed goods and the stuff you don't use, you have a clearer grasp of what you need to start fresh with a well-stocked pantry. Use the list in this article or get a printable version here. You may use this as a shopping list next time you go to the supermarket or order your food. Put a tick next to the goods you already have. From there, determine which goods you're going to add to your shopping list.

- Healthy Pantry Staples

Here's the list of healthy pantry necessities! That being said, don't feel like you need to fill your pantry with everything on this list or purchase everything at once. Use this as a guide. Pick your favorites or edit the list to your own preferences. Start building up your pantry inventory throughout the following month, and replace key goods as you run out or become low.

Dry Goods
Rolled oats
Quinoa Rice Beans (chickpeas, black, cannellini, etc)
Lentils
Pasta (enjoy Jovial brown rice, Banza, or lentil pasta)
Pasta sauce
Tomatoes (diced, roasted, paste)
Tomato sauce
Vegetable stock or broth
Salmon & tuna (wild-caught, canned)
Salsa
Nutritional yeast

Canned coconut milk
Coffee
Matcha
Herbal tea
Collagen peptides
Plant-based protein powder

Cooking Oils
Avocado oil
Avocado oil spray
Coconut oil
Extra virgin olive oil

Basic Herbs & Spices
Sea salt Black pepper
Basil Bay leaves
Cayenne Pepper Chili powder
Cinnamon
Crushed red pepper flakes
Cumin
Curry powder
Garlic powder
Ground ginger
Nutmeg
Paprika/Smoked paprika

Turmeric
Oregano

Pantry Freezer Staples
Bread (keeps your bread fresh longer!)
Cauliflower rice (Trader Joe's) Cauliflower gnocchi
(Trader Joe's)
Fruit (blueberries, raspberries, bananas, etc)
Vegetables
Veggie Burgers (Sunfoods, Amy's or Hillary's)
Shrimp Salmon

Longer - Lasting Produce
Acorn squash Apple Beets
Butternut squash
Cabbage
Carrots
Cauliflower Citrus Garlic
Onions
Parsnips
Pomegranates
Potatoes
Spaghetti squash
Sweet potatoes

CHAPTER FOUR

BUILDING A HEALTHY KITCHEN

Creating a healthy kitchen takes more than simply stocking it with nutritious goods. It also covers concerns for food preparation, cooking procedures, and general kitchen habits. Here are some strategies for establishing a healthy kitchen:

Stock Up on Nutrient-Rich Foods

Choose a range of fresh fruits and veggies.

Include whole grains such as brown rice, quinoa, and whole wheat.

Incorporate healthy fats from sources like avocados, almonds, and olive oil.

Minimize Processed Foods

Limit the presence of processed and packaged foods heavy in added sugars, salt, and harmful fats.

Read food labels to uncover hidden ingredients and preservatives.

Meal Preparation and Planning

- Plan meals in advance to maintain a balanced diet.

- Prepare and prepare healthful snacks for fast access.
- Cook in batches to have wholesome meals easily accessible throughout the week.

Choose Smart Cooking Methods
- Opt for baking, grilling, steaming, and sautéing over frying.
- Use herbs and spices for flavor instead of excessive salt.
- Experiment with various cooking ways to boost flavor without sacrificing nutrients.
- Invest in Quality Cookware
- Choose non-toxic cookware materials like stainless steel or cast iron.
- Avoid using non-stick cookware with possibly hazardous coatings.

Mindful Eating Environment
- Create a comfortable and appealing dining setting to encourage mindful eating.
- Limit distractions during meals, such as television or technological gadgets.

Proper Storage Practices
- Store perishable things at optimum temperatures to avoid spoiling.

- Use airtight containers to protect the freshness of fruits, vegetables, and leftovers.

Hygiene and Sanitation

- Maintain cleanliness in your kitchen to avoid foodborne diseases.
- Wash hands and surfaces routinely, particularly after handling raw meat or poultry.

Stay Hydrated

- Keep a water filter or water dispenser in the kitchen for convenient access to clean water.
- Limit sugary beverages and flavor water, herbal teas, or infused water.

Waste Reduction

- Reduce food waste by keeping leftovers.
- Compost kitchen wastes to lessen environmental effects.

Educate Yourself

- Stay educated on nutrition and healthy eating standards.
- Experiment with fresh recipes and cooking methods to keep meals entertaining and wholesome.

Building a healthy kitchen is a continuous effort that requires making mindful decisions about the foods you bring in, how you cook them, and the general setting in which you consume meals.

Essence of a Healthy Kitchen

Creating a healthy kitchen is crucial to fostering overall well-being, as it serves as the center of dietary decisions and food preparation in a home. The heart of a healthy kitchen is cultivating an atmosphere that fosters good eating habits and supports a balanced lifestyle. Here are crucial factors to consider while nurturing the essence of a healthy kitchen:

1. Whole, Nutrient-Rich Foods:
   - Prioritize entire foods such as fruits, vegetables, whole grains, lean meats, and healthy fats.
   - Minimize processed and highly refined items, since they generally include additional sugars, preservatives, and harmful fats.

2. Organized and Accessible Layout
   - Arrange your kitchen in a manner that makes healthy options more accessible. Keep fresh goods visible and within easy reach.
   - Organize your cupboard and refrigerator to eliminate clutter and make it simpler to access healthful foods.

3. Proper Kitchen Tools:
- Invest in kitchen gear that makes it simple to create nutritious meals, such as a sharp knife, cutting boards, and excellent cookware.
- Consider tools like blenders and food processors for producing homemade sauces, smoothies, and other nutritional meals.

4. Limited Processed Foods
- Minimize the presence of processed and convenience foods high in sugars, sodium, and unhealthy fats.
- Opt for homemade alternatives to control ingredients and nutritional content.

5. Hydration Station
- Keep water easily accessible in the kitchen. Consider infusing water with fruits and herbs for added flavor.
- Limit sugary drinks and prioritize water as the main beverage choice.

6. Mindful Eating Environment
- Create a pleasant dining space that encourages mindful eating.
- Avoid distractions like excessive screen time during meals and savor the flavors and textures of your food.

7. Storage Solutions

- Use storage containers to keep leftovers and meal-prepped items.
- Store healthful snacks like nuts, seeds, and cut-up veggies for quick access.

8. Nutrition Education

- Stay knowledgeable about nutrition to make intelligent eating choices.
- Encourage family members to learn about the nutritional worth of various foods and include them in meal planning.

9. Culinary Creativity

- Experiment with fresh recipes and cooking techniques to keep meals interesting and pleasurable.
- Explore a range of herbs and spices to improve tastes without depending on excessive salt or harmful condiments.

10. Cultural and Personal Adaptations

- Incorporate ethnic and personal culinary preferences into your healthy kitchen.
- Adapt healthy recipes to fit your taste and traditions, making it more likely to keep a balanced and pleasurable diet.

11. Regular Maintenance

- Regularly clean and arrange your kitchen to create a comfortable cooking environment.
- Discard old or harmful goods, preserving only those that contribute to a wholesome lifestyle.

By embracing these concepts, a healthy kitchen becomes a setting that not only enables the preparation of nutritional meals but also supports good attitudes towards food, supporting a holistic approach to well-being.

GLUTEN-FOOD

Gluten is a group of proteins present in wheat, barley, rye, and their derivatives. It has a critical function in supplying elasticity to dough, helping it rise and hold its form. Gluten is composed of two primary proteins: glutenin and gliadin. While gluten is a mainstay in many traditional dishes, it may pose health difficulties for persons with celiac disease, wheat allergy, or non-celiac gluten sensitivity.

Foods Containing Gluten:

Wheat-Based Products:

Bread: Most traditional bread is produced from wheat flour.

Pasta: Commonly produced from durum wheat semolina.

Cereal: Many morning cereals include wheat or wheat by-products.

Baked Goods:

Cakes, biscuits, muffins, and pastries commonly use wheat flour.

Pies with crusts prepared using conventional flour.

Processed Foods:

Many processed meals, such as soups, sauces, and gravies, may utilize wheat as a thickening ingredient.

Processed meats, such as sausages and deli meats, may include wheat-based fillers or binders.

Beer and Malt-Based Beverages:

Most traditional beers include barley, which is a gluten-containing grain.

Malt drinks and some ciders may potentially contain gluten.

Barley and Rye Products:

Barley-based items such as malt vinegar, barley malt extract, and various soups.

Rye bread and other rye-based meals.

Gluten-free food

A gluten-free diet entails avoiding the protein gluten, which is present in wheat, barley, rye, and their derivatives. This dietary option is necessary for persons with celiac disease, wheat allergy, or non-celiac gluten sensitivity. Adopting a gluten-free diet involves careful attention to food choices and a dedication to finding alternative products. Here's a guide to gluten-free foods:

Natural Gluten-Free Foods

- Fruits and Vegetables: Fresh fruits and vegetables are inherently gluten-free and supply crucial vitamins and minerals.

Incorporate a vibrant diversity into your diet.

- Meat and Poultry: Unprocessed meats, such as beef, chicken, turkey, and fish, are gluten-free.

Choose fresh cuts to reduce the danger of additional gluten-containing substances.

- Fish and Seafood: Most fish and seafood in their natural form are gluten-free.

Check for extra marinades or breading.

- Dairy and Eggs: Plain dairy items, such as milk, cheese, yogurt, and eggs, are inherently gluten-free.

Be careful with flavored or processed dairy products, since they may contain gluten additions.

- Legumes and Pulses: Beans, lentils, chickpeas, and other legumes are good sources of protein and fiber and are gluten-free.

Use them in soups, stews, salads, or as a meat alternative.

- Nuts and Seeds: Nuts and seeds, in their natural condition, are gluten-free.

Almonds, walnuts, chia seeds, flaxseeds, and sunflower seeds are popular alternatives.

- Gluten-Free Grains: Quinoa, rice, maize, millet, sorghum, and buckwheat are naturally gluten-free cereals.

Gluten-free oats may be ingested by people who tolerate them.

- Gluten-Free Flours: Almond flour, coconut flour, rice flour, chickpea flour, and sorghum flour are diverse gluten-free options for baking.
- Gluten-Free Pasta: Various gluten-free pasta varieties are available, manufactured from rice, maize, quinoa, or legumes.

- Gluten-Free Breads: Look for bread prepared from gluten-free flour such as rice, almond, or coconut flour.

Some companies provide gluten-free bread options in the market.

Gluten-Free Snacks: Popcorn, rice cakes, corn chips, and gluten-free crackers are snack alternatives without gluten.

- Gluten-Free Cereals: Choose cereals labeled gluten-free, made from rice, corn, or gluten-free oats.
- Gluten-Free Sauces & Condiments: Many sauces and condiments are naturally gluten-free, but it's crucial to check labels.

Tamari or gluten-free soy sauce can be used as alternatives.

Tips for a Successful Gluten-Free Lifestyle

- Label Reading: Individuals with gluten-related diseases must carefully examine food labels to uncover hidden sources of gluten.

Look for items labeled "gluten-free."

- Cross-Contamination: Be wary of cross-contamination in communal cooking environments.

Use separate utensils and cooking equipment for gluten-free dishes.

- Explore Gluten-Free Recipes: Experiment with gluten-free recipes to uncover great alternatives.

Many classic dishes may be altered using gluten-free ingredients.

- Gluten-Free Certification: Look for gluten-free certification markings on packaged items for further assurance.
- Consult with Professionals: Adopting a gluten-free lifestyle takes care, but with the plethora of naturally gluten-free foods and gluten-free alternatives available, it's quite possible to have a diversified, healthy, and tasty diet.

Recipes for Gluten-free Food

Gluten-free dishes may be tasty and enjoyable. Here are three gluten-free recipes for you to try:

1. Quinoa Salad with Overheated Veggies and Feta:

Ingredients:

1 cup quinoa, rinsed and cooked

2 cups mixed vegetables (e.g., cherry tomatoes, bell peppers, zucchini)

2 tablespoons olive oil

Salt and pepper to taste

1/2 cup crumbled feta cheese

Fresh

Fresh Herbs for garnishing

Instructions:

- Preheat the oven to 400°F (200°C).
- Toss the mixed veggies with olive oil, salt, and pepper. Roast in the oven for 20-25 minutes or until they are soft and slightly browned.
- In a large bowl, mix cooked quinoa and roasted veggies.
- Add crumbled feta cheese and stir gently.
- Garnish with fresh herbs before serving. Serve warm or cooled.

2. Grilled Chicken Lettuce Wraps:

Ingredients:

1 pound boneless, skinless chicken breasts
2 tablespoons gluten-free soy sauce
1 tablespoon olive oil
1 teaspoon honey
1 teaspoon minced garlic
Lettuce leaves (e.g., iceberg or butter lettuce)
Sliced veggies (carrots, cucumber, bell peppers) for stuffing

Instructions:

- In a bowl, mix together soy sauce, olive oil, honey, and minced garlic to make the marinade.
- Macerate chicken breasts in the mixture for at least 30 minutes.
- Grill chicken until thoroughly done, approximately 6-8 minutes each side.
- Slice the grilled chicken into strips.
- Assemble lettuce wraps by arranging chicken pieces and chopped veggies within lettuce leaves.
- Serve with more gluten-free soy sauce or a dipping sauce of your choice.

3. Gluten-Free Banana Bread: **Ingredients**:

2 ripe bananas, mashed

1/3 cup melted coconut oil or butter

1/4 cup honey or maple syrup

1 teaspoon vanilla extract

2 eggs

1 3/4 cups gluten-free flour mix

1 teaspoon baking soda

1/4 teaspoon salt

1/2 cup sliced nuts or chocolate chips (optional)

Instructions:

- Preheat the oven to 350°F (175°C). Grease a loaf pan.
- In a large bowl, combine mashed bananas, melted coconut oil or butter, honey or maple syrup, vanilla extract, and eggs.
- In a separate dish, mix together gluten-free flour, baking soda, and salt.
- Combine wet and dry components until just combined. Wrap in nuts or chocolate chips if you are using it.
- Put the batter into the already made loaf pan and level the top.

- Bake for at least 50-60 minutes or until a toothpick injected into the middle comes out smooth.
- You can cut it when the banana bread is cool.

CHAPTER FIVE

FRESH FOOD FAST

"Fresh Food Fast" symbolizes a modern and contemporary approach to sustaining our bodies with fresh, nutritious meals in a time-efficient way. In a world where tight schedules sometimes lead to fast-food choices that may compromise health, the notion of "Fresh Food Fast" strives to rethink the way we view short meals.

The core of this method rests in emphasizing fresh, complete foods that not only supply important nutrients but also contribute to a fulfilling and delectable culinary experience. It highlights the accessibility and practicality of including fruits, vegetables, lean meats, and whole grains in our everyday meals without losing nutritious value.

One of the primary benefits of "Fresh Food Fast" is its compatibility with a balanced and mindful eating philosophy. By selecting minimally processed meals, consumers may leverage the advantages of natural tastes and textures, encouraging fullness and lowering the temptation for less healthy options. Additionally, the brilliant colors and different tastes of fresh foods improve the whole sensory experience, making meals more delightful and rewarding.

The push towards "Fresh Food Fast" also corresponds with wider cultural movements toward sustainability and environmental conscience. Local, seasonal food not only tends to be fresher but also minimizes the carbon impact associated with shipping and long-term storage. Embracing this method not only boosts personal health but also supports local agriculture and encourages a more eco-friendly lifestyle.

In a world where time is frequently a limiting issue, "Fresh Food Fast" provides a practical answer to the difficulty of keeping a balanced diet. With the correct planning, preparation, and a focus on nutrient-dense options, people may manage their hectic lives while prioritizing their well-being. By fostering a culture that values fresh, quality products cooked with quickness, "Fresh Food Fast" becomes a cornerstone for a sustainable and health-conscious approach to contemporary life.

HEALTHY SNACKS

Healthy snacks serve an important role in sustaining overall well-being, offering a source of sustained energy between meals and contributing to a balanced diet. These snacks not only satiate hunger but also give us an opportunity to add necessary nutrients to our regular diet. Here are some crucial considerations and strategies for adding nutritious snacks to your routine:

- Nutrient Density: Opt for foods that carry a nutritious punch. Choose alternatives rich in vitamins, minerals, and other critical nutrients. Fresh fruits and vegetables, nuts, seeds, and whole grains are fantastic alternatives that give a broad variety of health advantages.

- Portion Control: While snacks are a crucial component of a balanced diet, it's essential to exercise in moderation. Pay attention to portion proportions to prevent overeating and to ensure that your snack adds to, rather than hinders, your overall nutritional objectives.

- Balance of Macronutrients: Aim for snacks that contain a balance of macronutrients, including carbs, proteins, and healthy fats. This equilibrium helps maintain energy

- levels, promotes satiety, and supports numerous biological processes.
- Hydration: Consider hydrating foods, such as water-rich fruits like watermelon or cucumber. Staying well-hydrated is vital for general health, and certain snacks may add to your regular fluid consumption.
- Preparation and Planning: Plan your snacks ahead of time to prevent grabbing for less healthy alternatives when hunger hits. Having a selection of healthful snacks readily accessible might make it simpler to make good choices throughout the day.
- Snacking on unprocessed Foods: Choose minimally processed, unprocessed foods as snacks. Examples include Greek yogurt with berries, a handful of almonds, sliced veggies with hummus, or a piece of whole-grain bread with avocado. These selections include a balance of nutrients and are often lower in added sweets and harmful fats.
- Mindful Eating: Practice mindful eating by enjoying your snacks and paying attention to hunger and fullness signs. Avoid distractions, such as electronics, and take the time to absorb the tastes and textures of your food.

- Diverse Options: Keep a range of nutritious snacks available to reduce boredom and to guarantee that you obtain a wide spectrum of nutrients. Rotate between various fruits, vegetables, nuts, and seeds to make snacking both fun and nutritionally varied.

By making deliberate choices and including a range of nutrient-dense snacks in your daily routine, you may promote your overall health and well-being while gratifying your taste senses.

FOOD FREEDOM

Food independence is a notion that incorporates the idea of establishing a healthy and balanced relationship with food, enabling people to make educated and conscious choices that match their personal tastes, health objectives, and cultural influences. It goes beyond basic dietary rules and limits, stressing the significance of enjoying food while fostering total well-being. Here are several major features of food freedom:

- Mindful Eating: Food freedom supports mindful eating, which means being completely present and attentive throughout

- meals. This practice helps people build a deeper connection with their bodies, detecting hunger and fullness signals, and relishing the tastes and textures of food.
- Intuitive Eating: Intuitive eating is a basic tenet of food independence, stressing the necessity of listening to the body's natural cues for hunger and contentment. This method fosters a non-restrictive attitude towards food and encourages people to trust their bodies to regulate their eating habits.
- Diverse and Inclusive Choices: dietary freedom encourages variety in dietary choices and acknowledges that there is no one-size-fits-all approach to nutrition. It encourages consumers to sample a broad variety of cuisines, including ethnic, seasonal, and personal tastes.
- Balanced and Flexible Approach: Rather than following rigorous diets or restrictive guidelines, food freedom advocates a balanced and flexible approach to eating. It understands that occasional excesses or diversions from a schedule are a normal component of a healthy relationship with food.

- Emotional Well-being: Food freedom understands the emotional components of eating and encourages people to create a healthy and loving connection with food. This involves comprehending and handling emotional triggers connected with eating without judgment.

- Education and Awareness: Food independence requires being knowledgeable about nutritional choices and knowing the influence of food on overall health. However, it encourages people to utilize this information as a tool for making empowered choices rather than developing a restricted worldview.

- Body Positivity: Embracing food freedom typically corresponds with the concepts of body positivity. It fosters self-acceptance and admiration for one's physique, concentrating on general well-being rather than adhering to cultural ideals of beauty.

- Pleasant Eating: Food freedom supports the concept that eating should be a pleasant and delightful activity. It helps people to find

- enjoyment in their meals, developing a positive attitude towards food that benefits both physical and emotional well-being.

By accepting the concept of food independence, people may build a healthy relationship with food that acknowledges their particular needs and tastes. This method develops a feeling of empowerment, autonomy, and pleasure in the act of eating, leading to a sustainable and rewarding lifestyle.

CONCLUSIONS

In conclusion, adopting a diet rich in nutritious foods is a vital step towards reaching and sustaining overall well-being. The multiple advantages associated with having a balanced and nutrient-dense diet extend beyond physical health, impacting mental clarity, emotional stability, and long-term vitality. By emphasizing fresh fruits, vegetables, whole grains, lean proteins, and vital fats, people may reinforce their immune systems, promote normal organ function, and lower the risk of chronic illnesses. Moreover, the good influence on energy levels, emotions, and cognitive function emphasizes the fundamental relationship between nutrition and holistic health.

Making educated decisions about the foods we eat not only benefits our own health but also leads to a more sustainable and ecologically conscientious lifestyle. Through mindful eating habits, we may cultivate a better understanding of the delicate link between our food choices and the larger ecology. As we understand the relevance of nutrition as a cornerstone of well-being, let us embrace the transformational potential of healthy food to pave the path to a full and meaningful life.